DIVERTICULITIS DIET COOKBOOK

Gut-Friendly Recipes For Symptom Relief And Digestive Health With Easy, Low-Fiber, Anti-Inflammatory Meal Plan

DR ELIAN GRIFFIN

Copyright © [Elian Griffin] [2024]. All rights reserved.

Without the publisher's prior written consent, no portion of this publication may be copied, distributed, or transmitted in any way, including by photocopying, recording, or other mechanical or electronic means, with the exception of brief quotations used in all critical reviews.

DISCLAIMER

The nutritional recommendations and recipes in this book are meant solely for informative reasons. They are not meant to replace the counsel, diagnosis, or care of a qualified medical expert. If you have any doubts about a medical condition or dietary requirements, you should always see your physician or another trained healthcare expert.

All reasonable efforts have been taken by the author and publisher to ensure that the information contained in this book is correct as of the date of publication. Recommendations may alter, though, as medical knowledge is always changing. When using any of the recipes or instructions found here, the user assumes all liability and assumes no risk, whether personal or otherwise. People who have certain dietary requirements or medical issues should speak with a healthcare provider for personalized guidance. The given recipes are only ideas; you may need to adjust them to suit your own nutritional needs, tastes, and tolerances.

When you use this book, you agree to release the publisher, the author, and their representatives from any liability for any claims, damages, liabilities, costs, or expenditures resulting from your use of the book.

TABLE OF CONTENTS

CHAPTER ONE 11
DIVERTICULITIS DIET INTRODUCTION 11
- IMPORTANCE OF MANAGING DIVERTICULITIS DIET 11
- HOW YOU CAN USE THIS COOKBOOK TO HELP 12
- ADVICE FOR EFFICIENT MEAL PLANNING 13

CHAPTER TWO 15
COMPREHENDING DIVERTICULITIS 15
- DIVERTICULITIS OVERVIEW 15
- REASONS AND SIGNS 16
- DIET IS IMPORTANT FOR TREATMENT 17
- OFTEN HELD MYTHS REGARDING DIVERTICULITIS 18
- THE EFFECTS OF DIET ON SYMPTOMS 19

CHAPTER THREE 21
CRUCIAL ELEMENTS FOR THE TREATMENT OF DIVERTICULITIS 21
- FIBER AND ITS FUNCTION 21
- THE VALUE OF DRINKING WATER 22
- GOOD FATS VERSUS BAD FATS 23
- SOURCES OF PROTEIN IN A BALANCED DIET 24
- MICRONUTRIENTS: WHAT THEY OFFER 25

CHAPTER FOUR 27
MEAL PLANNING FOR DIVERTICULITIS 27
- FORMULATING A WELL-BALANCED MEAL PLAN 27
- ESSENTIAL INGREDIENTS FOR A DIVERTICULITIS-FRIENDLY SHOPPING LIST 29
- MEAL PREP TECHNIQUES 30

- BUDGET-FRIENDLY CHOICES 31

BREAKFASTS RECIPES FOR DIGESTIVE HEALTH 33
- IDEAS FOR FIBER-RICH BREAKFASTS 33
- SMOOTHIES: A LOOK AT THEIR ADVANTAGES 34
- RECIPES FOR OATS OVERNIGHT 35
- OPTIONS FOR LOW-FAT BREAKFASTS 36
- ADDING PROBIOTICS 37

RECIPES FOR LUNCH AND DINNER 39
- RECIPES FOR HIGH-FIBER SALADS 39
- WHOLE GRAIN DINNERS 40
- OPTIONS FOR LEAN PROTEIN 42
- OPTIONS FOR VEGETARIANS AND VEGANS 43
- ONE-POT DINNERS FOR SIMPLE COOKING 45

SIDES AND SNACKS 47
- HEALTHY SNACK SUGGESTIONS 47
- RECIPES FOR HANDMADE TRAIL MIX 48
- SIDE DISHES MADE WITH VEGETABLES 49
- RECIPES FOR HEALTHFUL DIPS 50
- SIMPLE AND QUICK SNACK ASSEMBLY 51

DRINK SELECTIONS 53
- THE VALUE OF HYDRATION 53
- HERB TEAS FOR A HEALTHY DIGESTIVE SYSTEM 54
- DRINKS THAT INCREASE NUTRIENT CONTENT 55
- INFUSIONS OF WATER 56
- STEER CLEAR OF DEHYDRATING BEVERAGES 56

CHAPTER FIVE 59
PARTICULAR EVENTS AND SOCIAL GET-TOGETHERS............................59
ORGANIZING A DIVERTICULITIS-FRIENDLY GATHERING.....................59
IDEAS FOR A POTLUCK 60
RECIPES FOR HEALTHFUL DESSERTS...61
DIGESTION OF ALCOHOL WITH DIVERTICULITIS 62
TIPS FOR EATING OUT 63
CHAPTER SIX 65
HANDLING OUTBURSTS AND TYPICAL FEARS..65
RECOGNIZING FOOD TRIGGERS 65
MANAGING PAINFUL DIGESTION 66
WHEN TO GET MEDICAL ADVICE..67
TECHNIQUES FOR STRESS MANAGEMENT 68
MODIFICATIONS TO LIFESTYLE FOR LONG-TERM MANAGEMENT......69
CHAPTER SEVEN 71
FREQUENTLY ASKED QUESTIONS OR FAQS..71
DIVERTICULITIS: WHAT IS IT? 71
HOW DOES DIVERTICULITIS RELATE TO DIET? 72
WHICH MEALS OUGHT TO BE AVOIDED IF I HAVE DIVERTICULITIS?..73
CAN I STILL HAVE DESSERTS AND SNACKS? 74
HOW CAN I MAKE A BALANCED MEAL PLAN?..................................75

ABOUT THE BOOK

The "Diverticulitis Diet Cookbook" is an invaluable resource for anyone attempting to navigate the challenges of managing diverticulitis with dietary strategies. Diverticulitis is a condition characterized by inflammation or infection of small pouches (diverticula) in the digestive tract. Dietary management is necessary to reduce symptoms and avoid flare-ups. It is important to comprehend the basic principles of this condition, including its causes, and symptoms, and dispelling common misconceptions about its management. The cookbook provides readers with a thorough understanding of how particular dietary decisions can greatly affect the severity of symptoms and overall health.

The focus of this cookbook is on vital nutrients that are crucial to the management of diverticulitis. Each nutrient is described with its unique benefits and suggested sources, ranging from the importance of hydration and choosing healthy fats and proteins to the critical role that fiber intake plays in promoting digestive health. The cookbook not only teaches readers but also walks them through effective meal-planning techniques so they can effortlessly incorporate these dietary principles into their everyday lives.

This cookbook is all about being practical, as you can see from its methodical approach to making balanced meal plans, which includes weekly menu planning advice, necessary shopping lists, and effective meal prep techniques. It accommodates a variety of dietary needs and price ranges, with recipes ranging from fiber-filled breakfast ideas and nutrient-dense smoothies to filling lunch and dinner options that feature lean proteins and whole grains.

In addition, the cookbook discusses the subtleties of snacking and side dishes, offering wholesome substitutes that enhance culinary diversity and support digestive health. The cookbook also delves into beverage options, emphasizing the importance of staying hydrated and providing energizing options such as herbal teas and water infusions that support digestive wellness.

In addition, the cookbook provides helpful guidance on managing flare-ups and common concerns, including identifying trigger foods, relieving digestive discomfort, and incorporating stress management techniques into daily routines for long-term health maintenance. It also offers practical advice on hosting diverticulitis-friendly events and navigating dining-out scenarios.

Thorough FAQ section answers frequently asked questions concerning diverticulitis and diet management, giving readers access to concise, fact-based responses. This cookbook combines practical application with nutritional knowledge to give people the tools they need to take charge of their health and lead happy, fulfilling lives.

CHAPTER ONE

DIVERTICULITIS DIET INTRODUCTION

IMPORTANCE OF MANAGING DIVERTICULITIS DIET

Diet is crucial in the management of diverticulitis because certain foods can either relieve symptoms or cause flare-ups. This cookbook emphasizes the value of a well-balanced diet that contains high-fiber foods to support regularity in the digestive system and prevent inflammation.

By emphasizing foods that support gut health, people may be able to decrease the frequency and intensity of diverticulitis attacks. Additionally, maintaining a healthy weight through diet can relieve pressure on the colon and reduce abdominal pain.

When people with diverticulitis know what foods to eat and what to avoid, it can greatly enhance their quality of life. This cookbook offers helpful advice on how to choose foods that are easy on the digestive system but still tasty and filling.

By adhering to these dietary guidelines regularly, patients can take control of their condition and possibly avoid the need for medication or surgery.

HOW YOU CAN USE THIS COOKBOOK TO HELP

This cookbook is a comprehensive tool for anyone looking to manage their diverticulitis through diet; it offers a range of tasty and nutrient-dense recipes that are easy on the stomach while still providing essential nutrients; each recipe is made with ingredients that support gut health and reduce the likelihood of causing symptoms to flare up; it also includes meal preparation tips, ingredient substitutions, and portion control, making it suitable for cooks of all skill levels.

In addition, the cookbook offers informative material on the fundamentals of a diverticulitis-friendly diet, enabling readers to make knowledgeable decisions regarding their eating patterns.

By implementing these recipes into their everyday routine, people can benefit from better overall health and comfort in their digestive systems. This pragmatic method guarantees that long-term management of diverticulitis through diet is not only successful but pleasurable as well.

ADVICE FOR EFFICIENT MEAL PLANNING

The diverticulitis diet requires careful planning to be implemented successfully. This cookbook provides helpful advice on how to plan meals that are easy to prepare, balanced, and nutritious. It highlights the importance of incorporating a variety of foods from different food groups, such as lean proteins, whole grains, fruits, and vegetables, to ensure adequate intake of fiber and nutritional balance.

By organizing meals in advance, people can avoid making impulsive decisions that could exacerbate their symptoms of diverticulitis.

The cookbook also offers advice on meal frequency and portion sizes, promoting moderate but regular eating to support digestive health.

It also recommends keeping a food diary to monitor symptoms and identify triggers, which can help customize meal planning to meet specific needs. By adhering to these meal planning strategies, people can minimize the negative effects of diverticulitis on daily life while also maintaining diet consistency and optimizing their management of symptoms.

CHAPTER TWO

COMPREHENDING DIVERTICULITIS

DIVERTICULITIS OVERVIEW

Symptoms of diverticulitis include fever, nausea, vomiting, and changes in bowel habits such as diarrhea or constipation. Diverticulitis is a condition that arises when small pouches, called diverticula, form in the walls of the colon and become inflamed or infected. Usually, these pouches develop when weak spots in the colon's muscular walls give way under pressure, such as from constipation or straining during bowel movements.

Diverticulitis must be understood in terms of how it affects the digestive system. It is important to manage and treat diverticulitis as soon as possible to avoid complications such as abscesses, colon perforations, or even widespread infection (peritonitis). Treatment options for diverticulitis often include antibiotics to fight infections and dietary modifications to promote healing and prevent future flare-ups. In severe cases, hospitalization and surgery may be required.

REASONS AND SIGNS

Diverticula are little pouches or bulges that can form in the walls of the colon. These pouches are caused by weak spots in the muscular layers of the colon, which allow small areas to balloon outward, especially where the blood vessels enter. A low-fiber diet can cause constipation and increase the pressure inside the colon, which over time causes the walls of the colon to develop these pouches. Eventually, these pouches become inflamed or infected, which is what causes diverticulitis.

Diverticulitis can present with a wide range of symptoms, but the most common ones are fever, nausea, vomiting, changes in bowel habits (constipation or diarrhea), and abdominal pain, especially on the lower left side. Diverticulitis pain is usually chronic and can get worse over time. Severe cases can result in complications like abscesses or colon perforations, which need to be treated right away.

Early diagnosis and effective management of diverticulitis depend on knowing its causes and symptoms.

DIET IS IMPORTANT FOR TREATMENT

Foods high in fiber, such as fruits, vegetables, whole grains, and legumes, should be regularly consumed to promote healthy digestion and prevent complications associated with diverticulitis. Diet plays a critical role in the treatment and management of diverticulitis. A high-fiber diet is especially important because it helps to keep stools soft and regular, reducing the risk of constipation and straining during bowel movements. This, in turn, helps prevent the formation of diverticula and reduces the likelihood of them becoming inflamed or infected.

Drinking lots of water throughout the day helps to soften stools and ease their passage through the colon. Avoiding certain foods, like seeds, nuts, and popcorn, which can get lodged in the diverticula and cause irritation, is also recommended during flare-ups of diverticulitis.

Understanding the importance of a balanced, high-fiber diet and staying hydrated is key to managing diverticulitis effectively and reducing the frequency and severity of symptoms.

OFTEN HELD MYTHS REGARDING DIVERTICULITIS

Several common misconceptions about diverticulitis can lead to mismanagement and confusion. One such myth is that eating foods like popcorn, nuts, and seeds can either cause or worsen symptoms. However, recent research indicates that there is no concrete evidence connecting these foods to the onset or exacerbation of diverticulitis; for the majority of people with diverticulosis (diverticula present but not inflamed), these foods are generally safe to eat and a vital source of nutrients.

Another myth is that diverticulitis is only brought on by emotional or stressful situations. Although stress can aggravate digestive problems in some people, it is not a direct cause of diverticulitis. Instead, low-fiber diets, which cause constipation and elevated colonic pressure, and the presence of diverticula themselves are the main causes of diverticulitis. By recognizing these causes, misconceptions can be avoided and attention can be directed toward effective management strategies, such as dietary modifications and medical intervention when needed, to relieve symptoms and avoid complications.

THE EFFECTS OF DIET ON SYMPTOMS

The management and alleviation of diverticulitis symptoms are largely dependent on diet. A high-fiber diet is important because it softens stools and encourages regular bowel movements, which lowers the pressure inside the colon that can cause diverticula to become inflamed. Fruits, vegetables, whole grains, and legumes are high in fiber and should be regularly consumed to maintain digestive health. Adequate hydration is also necessary to prevent constipation and guarantee the smooth passage of stools through the colon.

Diverticulitis patients can better manage their symptoms and enhance their overall quality of life by being aware of how their diet affects their symptoms. By focusing on a balanced diet rich in fiber and staying hydrated, patients can effectively manage their symptoms and improve their overall quality of life. Certain foods and beverages, such as spicy foods, caffeine, alcohol, and high-fat foods, can irritate the digestive system and worsen abdominal pain.

CHAPTER THREE

CRUCIAL ELEMENTS FOR THE TREATMENT OF DIVERTICULITIS

FIBER AND ITS FUNCTION

To effectively manage the symptoms of diverticulitis, fiber is an essential part of a diverticulitis diet. It is known to help with regular bowel movements and prevent constipation. Diverticulitis diets should include both soluble and insoluble fiber. Soluble fiber dissolves in water and forms a gel-like substance in the intestines, which helps to soften and ease the passage of stools. Insoluble fiber adds bulk to stools, which helps them move through the digestive tract and prevents constipation. When combined, these fibers support regularity and guard against complications like diverticulitis flare-ups.

When it comes to adding fiber to your diet, whole grains—like brown rice, oats, and whole wheat bread—are a great source of insoluble fiber, which helps to bulk up stools and encourage regular bowel movements. You should also include a lot of fruits and vegetables in your meals—apples, berries, broccoli, and spinach are just a few examples—as they are excellent sources of both soluble and insoluble fiber.

Legumes—like beans and lentils—are also high in fiber and can be added to soups, salads, or main dishes to increase your daily intake of fiber. By adding these foods to your diet regularly, you can support digestive health and effectively manage the symptoms of diverticulitis.

THE VALUE OF DRINKING WATER

To ensure you're adequately hydrated, aim to drink 8-10 cups of water per day, or more if you're physically active or experiencing symptoms like diarrhea. Water plays a crucial role in digestion and helps soften stools, making them easier to pass and reducing the risk of constipation. For those who have diverticulitis, staying hydrated is especially important during flare-ups to prevent complications and support the healing process.

Water also helps flush toxins from the body and maintains normal bowel function, which is essential to preventing diverticulitis symptoms from getting worse.

Apart from water, you can also drink more herbal teas, broths, and fresh fruits and vegetables like watermelon and cucumbers. Avoid drinking too much alcohol and caffeinated drinks, as these can cause dehydration and upset the digestive tract. By making drinking plenty of water a daily habit, you can also help maintain healthy digestion, effectively treat the symptoms of diverticulitis, and enhance your overall health.

GOOD FATS VERSUS BAD FATS

To manage diverticulitis and preserve general health, it is important to choose the right fats. Monounsaturated and polyunsaturated fats, which are found in foods like avocados, nuts, seeds, and olive oil, are good for lowering inflammation and promoting heart health. They can also help improve blood vessel function and lower cholesterol, which is important for diverticulitis sufferers who may be at higher risk of cardiovascular disease. On the other hand, unhealthy fats, like saturated and trans fats, should be limited to prevent aggravating diverticulitis symptoms.

Make thoughtful food choices and prioritize healthy fats in your diet to support digestive health, manage inflammation, and promote overall well-being. To add healthy fats to your diet, use olive oil for cooking and salad dressings, eat nuts and seeds as a snack, and use avocados in salads or as a spread on whole-grain toast. Fatty fish, such as salmon and trout, are also excellent sources of omega-3 fatty acids, which have anti-inflammatory properties and can support overall health. The use of fried foods, processed snacks, and fatty cuts of meat, which are high in unhealthy fats, can exacerbate the symptoms of diverticulitis.

SOURCES OF PROTEIN IN A BALANCED DIET

Lean meats, such as chicken, turkey, and fish, are lower in saturated fats and easier to digest; plant-based proteins, like beans, lentils, and tofu, are also excellent choices; they provide fiber and essential nutrients without the saturated fat content of animal proteins. Including a variety of protein sources in your diet ensures you're getting essential amino acids and supporting overall health. Protein is essential for maintaining muscle mass, supporting immune function, and promoting healing, especially for individuals managing diverticulitis.

Greek yogurt and cottage cheese are also good sources of protein and can be enjoyed as snacks or added to smoothies for extra nutrition. Processed meats like bacon and sausage are high in saturated fats and sodium and may increase inflammation and worsen symptoms of diverticulitis. To incorporate protein into your meals, think about having grilled or baked chicken or fish as a main dish, adding beans or lentils to soups and salads, or enjoying tofu stir-fried with vegetables.

MICRONUTRIENTS: WHAT THEY OFFER

A variety of fruits, vegetables, whole grains, and lean proteins ensures you're getting a range of micronutrients that support digestive health and overall well-being.

Micronutrients, including vitamins and minerals, play essential roles in supporting overall health and managing diverticulitis. Key micronutrients for digestive health include vitamin C, which supports immune function and aids in wound healing, and vitamin D, which helps maintain bone health and may have anti-inflammatory effects. Minerals like magnesium are also important for muscle function and nerve health, while zinc supports immune function and wound healing.

To increase your consumption of micronutrients, try to include a variety of colors in your meals; for instance, oranges and strawberries are high in vitamin C, while leafy greens like spinach and kale are high in vitamin K and magnesium. You can also add essential minerals to your diet, such as zinc and magnesium, by incorporating nuts, seeds, and whole grains like quinoa and brown rice.

CHAPTER FOUR

MEAL PLANNING FOR DIVERTICULITIS

FORMULATING A WELL-BALANCED MEAL PLAN

A well-balanced meal plan for diverticulitis should emphasize foods high in fiber that are easy on the digestive tract. To begin, include high-fiber fruits like apples, berries, and pears, which supply vital vitamins and minerals in addition to their fiber content. Add extra fiber and nutrients to vegetables like spinach, kale, and broccoli.

Whole grains like oatmeal, brown rice, and whole wheat bread are great sources of soluble fiber that help with regular bowel movements and lessen the symptoms of diverticulitis.

Lean meats, poultry, and fish are good sources of protein that are low in inflammatory agents. Sources of healthy fats, such as avocado, nuts, and olive oil, can help maintain a healthy balance of gut bacteria, which is important in managing symptoms of diverticulitis.

Yogurt and other foods high in probiotics can help maintain a healthy balance of gut bacteria. By incorporating these foods into your meals and snacks throughout the day, you can create a well-rounded meal plan that promotes overall wellness and digestive comfort.

To effectively plan a weekly menu for diverticulitis, it is important to find safe, enjoyable recipes that include foods that are recommended. To start, choose ingredients that can be used for a variety of meals, such as quinoa, which is a nutritious base. Plan meals that include cooked vegetables, like squash, carrots, and zucchini, as they are easier to digest when steamed or roasted. You can also prepare soups and stews using low-fat broth, and you can add fiber-rich legumes, like lentils or chickpeas, for extra protein and fullness.

Plan and mix up your menu to enjoy tasty meals that support digestive health and ease the symptoms of diverticulitis. Add a variety of flavors and textures to keep meals interesting while making sure they meet your dietary needs. Use anti-inflammatory herbs and spices, such as turmeric, ginger, and garlic, to enhance taste and digestive benefits. Balance your intake of fiber across meals, aiming for gradual increases to prevent discomfort.

ESSENTIAL INGREDIENTS FOR A DIVERTICULITIS-FRIENDLY SHOPPING LIST

Creating a thorough shopping list guarantees you have the necessary supplies on hand for wholesome meals. Begin by assembling a large supply of fresh fruits and vegetables, emphasizing high-fiber options like berries, leafy greens, and cruciferous vegetables; select whole grains, such as brown rice, quinoa, and oats, which offer fiber and support regular digestion; and include lean proteins, such as turkey, chicken breast, and fish, selecting fresh or frozen products that don't need additional sauces or preservatives.

Add probiotics-rich dairy products like low-fat yogurt and cheese; add nuts, seeds, and olive oil for healthy fats that support reducing inflammation and promoting overall comfort in the digestive system; buy herbs and spices like cinnamon, parsley, and basil to add flavor to meals without adding too much salt or sugar; and make your grocery shopping trips more efficient by organizing these necessities into a shopping list that will guarantee you have everything you need to prepare healthy meals that support your management of diverticulitis.

MEAL PREP TECHNIQUES

To make daily eating routines easier, try batch cooking and portioning meals. To start, make big batches of high-fiber grains, like brown rice or quinoa, which can be used as a base for a variety of dishes throughout the week. Cook lean proteins, like baked fish or grilled chicken, and cook each portion separately for easy reheating. Wash and chop fresh produce ahead of time and store it in airtight containers so you can quickly access it when assembling meals.

Use slow cookers or instant pots to make low-fat soups and stews; add veggies and legumes for extra fiber and nutrients; label and store prepared ingredients in the refrigerator for quick meal assembly; this will cut down on cooking time and ease your hectic schedule. By following these meal prep tips, you can keep your diverticulitis diet consistent while guaranteeing well-balanced nutrition and comfortable digestion all week long.

BUDGET-FRIENDLY CHOICES

When following a budget-friendly diverticulitis diet, you should prioritize inexpensive ingredients that don't sacrifice nutritional quality. You should buy whole grains like oats and whole wheat pasta in bulk, which give you long-lasting energy and essential fiber without breaking the bank. You should also buy lean meat or poultry in larger portions and freeze any extra for later use to save even more money.

Look into plant-based protein sources like beans, lentils, and tofu, which are less expensive than animal proteins. When fresh produce isn't available, use canned or frozen fruits and vegetables to keep your diet varied without going over budget.

When cooking, use economical techniques like baking, steaming, or stir-frying to retain nutrients and flavor without going over budget. By sticking to these low-cost options, you can maintain a healthy diverticulitis diet without going over budget.

BREAKFASTS RECIPES FOR DIGESTIVE HEALTH

IDEAS FOR FIBER-RICH BREAKFASTS

Focusing on high-fiber breakfast ideas is critical for maintaining digestive health when following a diverticulitis diet. Whole grain cereals, such as oatmeal or bran flakes, are a great way to start the day. You can top them with fresh fruit, like bananas or berries, for extra fiber. Another great option is whole-grain toast with avocado, which provides healthy fats and fiber. You can also add flaxseeds or chia seeds to your yogurt bowls or smoothies to increase your intake of soluble fiber, which helps soften stools and ease bowel movements, decreasing the likelihood of flare-ups.

If you'd rather have a warm breakfast, try a vegetable omelet made with spinach, bell peppers, and tomatoes. Vegetables are a great source of fiber and important nutrients that support digestive health without causing discomfort. If you like to bake, try whole grain muffins or pancakes made with oat flour and topped with nuts or fruits.

These are homemade treats that are high in fiber and that you can customize to fit your diverticulitis diet goals. Throughout the day, stay hydrated as much as possible to aid in digestion and facilitate the movement of fiber through your digestive tract.

SMOOTHIES: A LOOK AT THEIR ADVANTAGES

A scoop of plain yogurt or a plant-based protein powder can enhance the smoothie's creaminess and provide probiotics, which are beneficial for gut health. Ground flaxseeds or chia seeds, which also contribute healthy fats and essential omega-3s, can also add extra fiber. Smoothies are versatile and convenient ways to incorporate nutrient-rich ingredients into your diverticulitis diet. They provide a concentrated source of vitamins, minerals, and fiber, all blended into a delicious and easy-to-digest drink.

Smoothies can be tailored to meet specific dietary requirements and nutritional needs. For example, if you like a thicker consistency, use frozen fruits or add a handful of oats for extra fiber.

If you need a low-sugar option, go for fruits like apples or berries, which have lower glycemic indexes. Smoothies are great for breakfast or as a snack in between meals, offering sustained energy without causing discomfort in the digestive tract. They can also help maintain hydration levels, which is especially useful during flare-ups.

RECIPES FOR OATS OVERNIGHT

For those who manage diverticulitis, overnight oats are a quick, easy, and nutrient-dense breakfast option that can be tailored to your taste buds and dietary needs. To begin, combine old-fashioned oats with a liquid (yogurt, almond milk, etc.) in a jar or container. Top with your favorite toppings (fresh fruits, nuts, seeds, or a drizzle of honey for sweetness), and let the oats absorb the liquid overnight to create a creamy, satisfying, and gentle-on-the-stomach breakfast.

Overnight oats can be made in batches and kept in the refrigerator for several days, making them a convenient grab-and-go option for busy mornings.

Try experimenting with different flavor combinations to find your favorite variation that supports your digestive health goals. If you're looking for a recipe that's high in fiber, try adding ingredients like chia seeds, which provide additional soluble fiber and omega-3 fatty acids. You can also add mashed bananas or applesauce for natural sweetness and added fiber content.

OPTIONS FOR LOW-FAT BREAKFASTS

Reducing the amount of fat in your breakfast is crucial for controlling the symptoms of diverticulitis and maintaining digestive health in general. Lean protein sources, like egg whites, turkey sausage, or Greek yogurt, offer vital nutrients without being fattening. Boiled or scrambled eggs combined with whole-grain toast or English muffins make a filling and well-balanced breakfast. Fruit salad with a dollop of low-fat cottage cheese or a low-fat milk or almond milk smoothie are lighter options that are easy on the stomach and can help avoid the discomfort that comes with eating high-fat foods.

Whole grain toast or oatmeal, for example, contains fiber that promotes healthy digestion. Cooking with baking, broiling, or steaming techniques instead of frying can help you consume less fat without sacrificing nutritional value. For a quick and healthy breakfast, try whole-grain cereal with skim milk and a serving of fresh fruit; this combination provides the fiber, vitamins, and minerals required to keep your digestive system regular. By selecting low-fat options and emphasizing nutrient-dense foods, you can maintain your digestive health while savoring tasty and filling breakfasts.

ADDING PROBIOTICS

Probiotics are important for gut health and are simple to include in your diverticulitis diet. One way to start your day is with a probiotics-rich food like plain Greek yogurt, which has live cultures that are good for your digestive system. You can add fresh fruit, nuts, or a drizzle of honey to make the yogurt taste better and have more nutrients. Another option is kefir, which is a dairy product that has been fermented and contains probiotics. You can eat kefir plain or blend it into smoothies for a creamy, tart breakfast treat.

To support long-term digestive health and overall well-being, if you enjoy baking, try making homemade sourdough bread using a natural fermentation process, which enhances probiotics content. If you prefer plant-based options, consider including fermented foods like sauerkraut or kimchi in your morning routine. These foods contain probiotics bacteria that support a healthy balance of gut flora and promote digestive wellness. Including probiotics in your breakfast can help maintain a diverse microbiome and reduce inflammation associated with diverticulitis. Whenever possible, aim to include probiotics-rich foods as part of a balanced diet.

RECIPES FOR LUNCH AND DINNER

RECIPES FOR HIGH-FIBER SALADS

For a diverticulitis diet, high-fiber salads are a must-have because they supply the nutrients needed without taxing the digestive system. Start with a base of leafy greens, like spinach, kale, or arugula, which are high in fiber and simple to digest. Top with a variety of colorful vegetables, like bell peppers, cucumbers, and tomatoes, for extra fiber, vitamins, and antioxidants. Add seeds and nuts, like slivered almonds or chia seeds, to increase the fiber content and give a delightful crunch. For a dressing, use a light mixture of olive oil and lemon juice; steer clear of dressings too creamy or heavy.

Fruits such as berries, apple slices, or orange segments can add a sweet and fiber-rich twist to your salads. These fruits are not only delicious but also a great source of vitamins and antioxidants. Legumes such as black beans or chickpeas are high in protein and fiber, adding substantialness to your salads.

You can also boost the fiber content of your salads with quinoa or a sprinkle of flaxseed to help improve digestive health.

Try experimenting with different textures and flavors to keep your salads interesting and varied. Roasted veggies, like sweet potatoes or carrots, can give your salad a warm, hearty element. Add whole grains, like bulgur or farro, for an extra fiber boost. Fresh herbs, like parsley, cilantro, or basil, can add a burst of flavor. A little avocado adds healthy fats and a creamy texture. These high-fiber salad recipes are delicious and versatile, so they're a great way to incorporate them into your diet.

WHOLE GRAIN DINNERS

For a simple yet nutritious meal, cook brown rice and combine it with steamed vegetables like broccoli, carrots, and peas. Add a lean protein source like grilled chicken or tofu to create a balanced meal that's easy on the digestive system. Whole-grain entrees are an excellent way to ensure a high-fiber diet, crucial for those managing diverticulitis. Start with versatile grains like brown rice, quinoa, or barley as the foundation for your meals. These grains are packed with fiber and essential nutrients, providing a hearty and satisfying base.

Whole grain risottos, made with farro or barley instead of Arborio rice, can also be a delightful option. Cook with vegetable broth, and add mushrooms, spinach, and a sprinkle of Parmesan cheese for a comforting, high-fiber dish. Or try whole wheat, spelled, or quinoa pasta for a fiber-rich alternative to traditional pasta.

Pair it with a variety of vegetables like zucchini, mushrooms, and bell peppers, sautéed in olive oil and garlic. Add a light tomato sauce or a pesto made from fresh basil and pine nuts for a tasty and healthful meal.

Try adding whole grains to international cuisines for a more exotic twist. For example, make a hearty barley and vegetable stew with tomatoes, carrots, celery, and your favorite herbs and spices. These whole-grain entrees not only support digestive health but also offer a world of flavors and textures to keep your meals exciting and nutritious. Prepare a quinoa-based tabbouleh with fresh parsley, mint, tomatoes, and cucumbers, dressed with lemon juice and olive oil.

OPTIONS FOR LEAN PROTEIN

A diverticulitis-friendly diet must include lean protein sources because they are easier to digest and less likely to irritate the digestive tract. Skinless poultry, like chicken or turkey, is an excellent source of lean protein; cook it by grilling, baking, or broiling it to maintain its health; season it with herbs like oregano, rosemary, or thyme to add flavor without adding a lot of sauce; and serve it with roasted or steamed vegetables and a serving of whole grains for a balanced meal.

Another great lean protein option is fish, which is high in omega-3 fatty acids that can help lower inflammation. Choose fish that is baked or grilled, and season it with a little lemon and dill to add flavor without adding extra fat. For a quick and easy lunch, try a tuna salad that is made with Greek yogurt instead of mayonnaise, mixed with diced celery, carrots, and mustard, and served on a bed of leafy greens or whole grain crackers.

Legumes—such as lentils, chickpeas, and black beans—are excellent plant-based protein options because they are high in protein and also contain a good amount of fiber. You can make a lentil stew with tomatoes, carrots, and celery for a filling and healthy meal, or you can make a chickpea and quinoa salad with diced cucumbers, tomatoes, and parsley that is dressed with olive oil and lemon juice. These lean protein options make sure you get the nutrients you need while adhering to a diet that promotes digestive health.

OPTIONS FOR VEGETARIANS AND VEGANS

There are plenty of vegetarian and vegan options that are high in fiber and essential nutrients for people with diverticulitis. To start, try grains that are versatile and can be used as a complete protein source, such as bulgur or quinoa, and then combine them with a variety of vegetables and legumes to make filling and healthy meals. For example, quinoa and black bean salad with corn, bell peppers, and a lime-cilantro dressing is a great option; add avocado for healthy fats and a creamy texture that goes well with the other ingredients.

Another great option is vegetable stir-fries, which are simple to tailor with your favorite vegetables. Tofu or tempeh can be used as a source of protein; they can be cooked in a light soy sauce or teriyaki glaze. Add colorful and nutrient-dense vegetables such as bell peppers, broccoli, and snap peas to create a vibrant dish. Serve over brown rice or whole grain noodles for a full meal. Top with chopped nuts or sesame seeds for extra fiber and nutrients.

In addition to being satisfying and easy to digest, soups and stews can also be substantial vegetarian and vegan options. For example, a lentil and vegetable stew simmered with tomatoes, carrots, and celery is a hearty and digestible meal. A curry made with chickpeas and spinach, cooked with coconut milk and spices like turmeric and cumin, is a flavorful and comforting dish.

These dishes can be made in large quantities and frozen for easy weekday meals.

ONE-POT DINNERS FOR SIMPLE COOKING

A chicken and vegetable rice pilaf, cooked with carrots, peas, and bell peppers, is a simple and delicious option. Season with herbs and a touch of olive oil for a dish that's both flavorful and easy on the digestive system. One-pot meals are ideal for those managing diverticulitis, offering simplicity and convenience while ensuring nutritious and balanced eating. Start with a base of whole grains like brown rice, quinoa, or barley, which cook well in a single pot and provide a solid fiber foundation. Combine with a variety of vegetables and lean proteins to create a complete meal.

Another great option is a one-pot lentil and vegetable stew, which is cooked with onions, garlic, bell peppers, and tomatoes. Season with chili powder, cumin, and paprika for a hearty and satisfying meal that's easy on the stomach. Combine lentils with diced tomatoes, carrots, celery, and spinach, and simmer with vegetable broth and your favorite herbs and spices. This meal is high in fiber and protein, making it both nutritious and filling. Squeeze lemon juice over the dish before serving to bring out the flavors.

Another quick and simple fix is to make one-pot pasta dishes. Use whole grain or gluten-free pasta and cook it with a variety of veggies, such as spinach, zucchini, and mushrooms. To keep the sauce light and easily digested, add a light tomato sauce or a broth-based sauce. Lean meats, such as ground turkey or chicken breast, or plant-based options, such as tofu or chickpeas, can be added for extra protein. These one-pot meals not only make cleanup easier but ensure you have a balanced, nutritious meal that supports your digestive health.

SIDES AND SNACKS

HEALTHY SNACK SUGGESTIONS

Finding satiating and low-fat snacks is essential to keeping a diverticulitis-friendly diet going. To support digestive health, look for high-fiber, low-fat snacks. Fresh fruits, such as berries, apples, and bananas, are great because of their fiber content and natural sweetness; pair them with a small serving of low-fat yogurt or cottage cheese for extra protein. Raw vegetables, such as carrot sticks, cucumber slices, and bell pepper strips, are also great because they provide fiber and important vitamins without making you feel uncomfortable.

When you're craving something more substantial, think about whole-grain snacks like rice cakes or whole wheat crackers, which are easy on the digestive tract and provide fiber. Nut butter like peanut or almond butter can be spread on whole-grain toast or combined with apple slices for a balanced snack that combines protein and fiber.

Stay away from snacks that are high in processed sugars or saturated fats, as these can aggravate the symptoms of diverticulitis. By selecting nutrient-dense snacks, you can effectively manage diverticulitis while maintaining a healthy diet.

RECIPES FOR HANDMADE TRAIL MIX

Making your trail mix lets you alter the components to suit your tastes and dietary requirements while keeping it diverticulitis-safe. To begin, use unsalted nuts like almonds, walnuts, and pecans, which offer protein and healthy fats without any added sodium. Next, add dried fruits like raisins, cranberries, or apricots for natural sweetness and fiber. Finally, add seeds like pumpkin or sunflower seeds to improve texture and flavor while providing important nutrients and crunch.

Once all ingredients are well combined, portion into small, resealable bags for easy on-the-go snacking throughout the day. Not only does homemade trail mix satisfy hunger, but it also provides essential nutrients needed to support digestive health and overall well-being, making it an ideal snack option for those with diverticulitis. For a savory twist, add whole-grain cereal or pretzel pieces to the mix. Season lightly with herbs like rosemary or thyme and a sprinkle of sea salt if desired.

SIDE DISHES MADE WITH VEGETABLES

Vegetable side dishes are a staple of a diverticulitis diet because they are high in fiber, vitamins, and minerals, and they are good for your digestive tract. Roasted vegetables, like carrots, broccoli, and cauliflower, are easy to prepare and can be flavored with herbs like garlic, thyme, or paprika. Steamed or sautéed leafy greens, like spinach or kale, are great because they are high in fiber and have a mild effect on the digestive system.

To make a satisfying side dish, try making a colorful stir-fry with bell peppers, zucchini, and snap peas; use a small amount of olive oil and season with herbs or low-sodium soy sauce to add flavor without sacrificing nutrients.

You can also make a fresh salad with mixed greens, cucumber, tomatoes, and avocado and dress it with a light vinaigrette dressing. Eating a balanced diet that promotes digestive health and effectively manages symptoms of diverticulitis can be achieved by including a variety of colorful vegetables in your meals.

RECIPES FOR HEALTHFUL DIPS

Healthy dip recipes are a great way to add some flavor and nutrients to your snacking while also supporting digestive health. Try dips made with Greek yogurt or low-fat sour cream as a base; these are higher in protein and lower in fat than traditional dips. To add some flavor, add fresh herbs like dill, parsley, or chives, and squeeze some lemon juice for brightness. Hummus, which is made from chickpeas and tahini, is another healthy option that provides plant-based protein and fiber.

Serve dips with raw vegetable sticks like celery, carrots, and cucumber for added fiber and crunch. Steer clear of dips high in saturated fats or sodium, as these can contribute to inflammation and discomfort. Instead, choose nutrient-dense ingredients and emphasize fresh flavors to enjoy delicious dips that support digestive health and improve your overall well-being. Ripe avocados make a satisfying and creamy alternative to guacamole, which is made with lime juice, garlic, and a small pinch of salt.

SIMPLE AND QUICK SNACK ASSEMBLY

Simple and high-nutrient snacks are essential for managing diverticulitis. Make grab-and-go snacks, such as pre-cut fruit and vegetable containers that are kept in your refrigerator for easy access. Wash and slice fruits, like melons, berries, and grapes, and store them in portioned containers for easy access all week. Similarly, chop up veggies, like bell peppers, sugar snap peas, and cherry tomatoes, to keep on hand for easy snacking.

For high-protein snacks, hard-boiled eggs or small portions of low-fat cheese or Greek yogurt make a satisfying snack that combines protein and fiber.

Alternatively, you can make your energy bars ahead of time, which are made of oats, nuts, seeds, and dried fruits bound together with a natural sweetener such as honey or maple syrup. These bars offer sustained energy and nutrients without the added ingredients of store-bought varieties. By setting aside a small amount of time for snack prep, you can be sure to have nourishing options on hand to effectively support your diverticulitis diet goals.

DRINK SELECTIONS

THE VALUE OF HYDRATION

Drinking enough water throughout the day supports the body's natural detoxification processes, which flush out toxins and promote healthy digestion.

It also helps prevent constipation, which is a common problem for people with diverticulitis. Hydration is essential for maintaining overall health, especially when managing conditions like these.

Drink 8 to 10 glasses of water a day, spread your water intake throughout the day instead of consuming large amounts at once, and watch the color of your urine—pale yellow indicates adequate hydration, while darker colors may indicate dehydration. Herbal teas and water-based foods, such as fruits and vegetables, also contribute to your overall fluid intake.

HERB TEAS FOR A HEALTHY DIGESTIVE SYSTEM

Because of their calming and digestive qualities, herbal teas are a great addition to a diverticulitis diet. Peppermint tea, for example, has a calming effect on the digestive tract and can help relieve symptoms like gas and bloating.

Chamomile tea has anti-inflammatory qualities that can lessen intestinal inflammation and discomfort related to diverticulitis. Ginger tea promotes digestion and can help with nausea and vomiting, which are common during flare-ups.

Herbal teas can be made by steeping 1-2 teaspoons of dried herbs or a tea bag in hot water for 5-10 minutes; strain and serve warm. Herbal teas can be consumed between meals or as part of a relaxation routine; if you need to sweeten, use honey or stevia instead of artificial sweeteners. Try experimenting with different herb combinations to see which ones work best for your digestive system.

DRINKS THAT INCREASE NUTRIENT CONTENT

Smoothies are a convenient and nutrient-dense option for people with diverticulitis. They offer vital vitamins, minerals, and fiber in an easily digestible form. To support healthy digestion and encourage regular bowel movements, use ingredients like spinach, kale, or other leafy greens rich in fiber.

Berries, which are low in fiber and high in antioxidants, can add flavor and essential nutrients without exacerbating symptoms.

Blend 1 cup leafy greens, 1 cup berries, 1 small banana, and 1 tablespoon ground flaxseed or chia seeds for extra fiber to make a diverticulitis-friendly smoothie; use water or low-fat yogurt as a base to achieve a smooth consistency; stay away from high-fiber fruits with seeds or skins that could irritate the digestive tract; drink smoothies slowly to facilitate digestion and avoid discomfort.

INFUSIONS OF WATER

Cucumber and mint infusions offer a cooling effect and aid in digestion; berries like strawberries or blueberries add a hint of sweetness and antioxidants; and fruits like lemon, lime, or oranges add a citrusy twist and vitamin C, an antioxidant that supports immune function and tissue repair, to water. Water infusions are a refreshing way to increase fluid intake while adding natural flavors without added sugars or calories.

To make water infusions, cut up fruits, vegetables, or herbs and place the pitcher in the fridge for a few hours to allow the flavors to infuse. Then, serve the chilled water over ice for a refreshing drink all day long. Try different combinations to find flavors that you enjoy and that will maintain the ideal level of hydration for you.

STEER CLEAR OF DEHYDRATING BEVERAGES

Alcohol should be limited or avoided as it can irritate the digestive tract and contribute to dehydration.

Sugary drinks like sodas and energy drinks provide empty calories and can exacerbate digestive symptoms. Caffeinated drinks like coffee and black tea should be avoided as they can act as a diuretic, increasing urine production and potentially leading to dehydration.

To maintain optimal hydration and effectively manage symptoms of diverticulitis, choose hydrating drinks such as water, herbal teas, and diluted fruit juices. Carefully read labels and select beverages without added sugars or artificial ingredients. Pay attention to how your body reacts to different drinks and make adjustments to your selections accordingly.

CHAPTER FIVE

PARTICULAR EVENTS AND SOCIAL GET-TOGETHERS

ORGANIZING A DIVERTICULITIS-FRIENDLY GATHERING

It takes careful planning to host a diverticulitis-friendly event so that everyone can eat delicious food without sacrificing their health. Start by choosing a range of high-fiber, low-fat foods that are easy on the digestive system, like fruits, vegetables, and whole grains. Add lean proteins, like grilled chicken or fish, which are easier to digest than fatty meats.

Make sure there are plenty of hydration options available, like infused water or herbal teas, to promote digestive health. Serve food in smaller portions to avoid overindulging, which can exacerbate symptoms. Finally, ask guests about their dietary preferences and restrictions so that everyone can enjoy delicious meals without compromising their health.

The secret to a successful diverticulitis-friendly event is to create a warm and inviting environment. Incorporate low-fiber options like cooked vegetables or mashed potatoes for those with more sensitive digestive systems. Use vibrant and inviting table settings with fresh flowers or simple centerpieces to enhance the dining experience. Provide clear labels for each dish, indicating ingredients and potential allergens, to help guests make informed choices. Encourage mindful eating by offering smaller plates and suggesting a slower eating pace to aid in digestion.

IDEAS FOR A POTLUCK

A diverticulitis-friendly potluck entails planning a range of appetizing and filling dishes that are easy on the digestive system and still delicious. To support digestive health, ask guests to bring fiber-rich salads made with leafy greens, beans, and whole grains. You can also think about serving a main course such as lightly seasoned grilled chicken or fish. For those who need more fiber without sacrificing flavor, consider serving vegetable skewers or roasted sweet potatoes. Finally, for those who want something refreshing and simple to digest for dessert, serve fresh fruit platters or yogurt parfaits.

You can enjoy a potluck that encourages well-being and shared culinary enjoyment among friends and family by creating a balanced potluck menu that offers something for everyone while supporting digestive wellness. Work with guests to avoid common trigger foods, like spicy dishes or heavy sauces, which can exacerbate symptoms. Provide serving utensils for each dish and encourage portion control to prevent overeating, which can strain the digestive system. Label each dish with ingredients and dietary information to help guests make informed choices.

RECIPES FOR HEALTHFUL DESSERTS

Diverticulitis-friendly desserts are made with ingredients that are easy on the digestive tract but still satisfy sweet tooth. Fruit-based desserts, such as baked apples or poached pears, offer natural sweetness and fiber. When baking, use whole-grain flour or oats to boost fiber without making you feel uncomfortable. Try lowering the fat content of recipes by using low-fat dairy or plant-based substitutes. Use natural sweeteners, such as honey or maple syrup, sparingly, taking into account each person's tolerance levels.

Experimenting with portion sizes and serving styles can encourage moderation and mindful eating habits. By incorporating nutritious ingredients and minimizing triggers, you can create delicious desserts that align with diverticulitis dietary guidelines and promote overall well-being. You can also enjoy and feel fulfilled when you find creative ways to indulge in desserts while supporting digestive wellness. For example, try making chia seed pudding with almond milk and fresh berries for a fiber-rich treat.

DIGESTION OF ALCOHOL WITH DIVERTICULITIS

Drinking alcohol while having diverticulitis means being mindful of potential triggers and consuming it in moderation to avoid discomfort.

Clear spirits, such as vodka or gin, combined with low-acid fruit juices or sparkling water, are lighter options. Sugary mixers and cocktails can exacerbate symptoms; instead, choose natural flavors. Drink no more than one or two glasses of alcohol at a time to reduce the negative effects on digestive health.

You can enjoy occasional drinks while supporting digestive health and well-being by being informed about your personal tolerance levels and potential triggers, keeping an eye on your symptoms, and avoiding excessive consumption, which can worsen digestive discomfort and dehydrate the body. When it comes to resting and recuperating from alcohol, choose days when you don't drink to promote overall wellness. When you socialize, let hosts or bartenders know about your dietary needs and preferences to ensure that options are in line with diverticulitis dietary guidelines.

TIPS FOR EATING OUT

To ensure a positive dining experience when dining out with diverticulitis, carefully consider menu options and preparation methods to avoid trigger foods and promote digestive comfort. Look up fiber-rich and low-fat options online, such as grilled lean meats, salads with dressing on the side, and steamed vegetables. Ask servers about substitutions of ingredients or methods of preparation to accommodate dietary restrictions and preferences. Share plates or order smaller portions to avoid overeating and lessen the strain on the digestive system.

You can make the most of your dining out experience with diverticulitis by selecting restaurants that offer flexible menus and friendly staff; choosing dishes that are mildly seasoned and steer clear of spicy or highly processed foods that may aggravate symptoms; drinking water or herbal teas throughout the meal to stay hydrated; engage in mindful eating by chewing food slowly and enjoying each bite to aid in digestion; schedule dining outings during slower times of the day to promote relaxation and reduce stress; and make educated choices and stand up for your dietary needs.

CHAPTER SIX

HANDLING OUTBURSTS AND TYPICAL FEARS

RECOGNIZING FOOD TRIGGERS

Once you've identified potential triggers, you should gradually eliminate them from your diet to see if symptoms improve. One of the most important things to do when managing diverticulitis through diet is to identify common trigger foods, which can include nuts, popcorn, seeds, and some raw vegetables like peppers or cucumbers that can aggravate flare-ups. It's important to observe how your body reacts to different foods as triggers vary from person to person.

To help regulate bowel movements without irritating, replace nuts and seeds with smooth nut milk or nut butter. Cook vegetables thoroughly to facilitate digestion.

Choose soluble fiber sources such as applesauce, oats, and peeled fruits. By taking proactive measures to manage trigger foods, you can lessen the frequency and intensity of diverticulitis symptoms and improve overall digestive health.

MANAGING PAINFUL DIGESTION

Diverticulitis-related digestive discomfort can be managed by following certain dietary and lifestyle guidelines. When symptoms are present, choose a low-fiber diet to temporarily rest the digestive system. Consume easily digested foods such as cooked fruits, soft meats, and refined grains. Drink plenty of water and herbal teas to stay hydrated and help prevent constipation, which is a common symptom of diverticulitis. Avoid alcohol and caffeine as they can irritate the digestive tract and exacerbate symptoms.

By implementing these strategies, you can effectively manage digestive discomfort associated with diverticulitis and support overall digestive wellness. Probiotics-rich foods, like yogurt or kefir, can also help alleviate discomfort. Over-the-counter medications, such as pain relievers or antispasmodics, can temporarily relieve cramping or abdominal pain.

However, make sure to consult your healthcare provider before using any medications, especially if you have other medical conditions or are taking other medications.

WHEN TO GET MEDICAL ADVICE

Effective management of diverticulitis requires knowing when to seek medical advice. If you have severe abdominal pain, fever, vomiting, or noticeable changes in your bowel habits, you should see a doctor right away. These symptoms may indicate complications like an infection or bowel obstruction, which need to be treated right away. If your symptoms worsen or continue even after you've changed your diet and taken care of yourself at home, you should see a doctor for additional assessment and treatment.

Regular visits to your physician are also essential, particularly if you have a medical history of diverticulitis or other digestive disorders. They can monitor your condition, offer advice on dietary modifications, and suggest necessary screenings or treatments. Proactive management and early intervention can help prevent complications and improve long-term outcomes for those who suffer from diverticulitis.

TECHNIQUES FOR STRESS MANAGEMENT

Stress reduction is essential for managing diverticulitis because stress can aggravate symptoms and cause flare-ups. Deep breathing, yoga, meditation, and other relaxation techniques can lower stress levels and enhance general well-being. Walking or swimming regularly can also help reduce stress and improve digestion. Finally, develop a regular sleep schedule to guarantee that you get enough sleep, as sleep deprivation can exacerbate symptoms and lead to stress.

If stress is hurting your mental health or daily life, consider speaking with a therapist or counselor. By implementing stress management techniques into your routine, you can help reduce the frequency and severity of diverticulitis symptoms, which will improve your overall quality of life.

Some enjoyable and relaxing activities to consider include gardening, reading, and spending time with loved ones.

MODIFICATIONS TO LIFESTYLE FOR LONG-TERM MANAGEMENT

Long-term management of diverticulitis requires a lifestyle change. To encourage regular bowel movements and prevent the progression of the disease, adopt a high-fiber diet rich in fruits, vegetables, whole grains, and legumes. Increase fiber intake gradually to avoid abrupt changes that could be uncomfortable. Stay hydrated throughout the day by drinking lots of water; this will support digestive health and help prevent constipation.

Aim for at least 30 minutes of moderate physical activity most days of the week, such as brisk walking, cycling, or strength training. Avoid smoking and limit alcohol consumption as these behaviors can exacerbate digestive issues and hinder recovery. Practice good bathroom habits by promptly responding to bowel urges and avoiding straining during bowel movements. Maintaining overall health and preventing complications from diverticulitis depend on regular exercise.

You can effectively control your diverticulitis symptoms and enhance your overall quality of life over time by implementing these lifestyle changes and adhering to a personalized management plan. Relaxation techniques are important for stress management and should be incorporated into your daily routine to prevent flare-ups.

CHAPTER SEVEN

FREQUENTLY ASKED QUESTIONS OR FAQS

DIVERTICULITIS: WHAT IS IT?

Diverticulitis is a disorder that causes small, bulging pouches in the digestive tract to become inflamed or infected. These pouches, also called diverticula, usually form in weak areas of the colon lining, particularly where blood vessels pass through the muscle layer. Symptoms of diverticulitis include fever, nausea, and changes in bowel habits. Severe cases of the infection may necessitate hospitalization and antibiotics.

Physical examinations, imaging tests (such as CT scans), and blood tests to confirm inflammation or infection in the diverticula are often used in the diagnosis of diverticulitis.

 Dietary modifications, such as a clear liquid diet for a short while to rest the digestive system, are then gradually added back in to promote regular bowel movements and prevent future flare-ups. Occasionally, medications and, very rarely, surgery, are required.

HOW DOES DIVERTICULITIS RELATE TO DIET?

A high-fiber diet is usually advised as it helps soften and add bulk to stools, making them easier to pass and reducing pressure on the colon walls. This can prevent the development of diverticula and decrease the likelihood of inflammation or infection. Whole grains, fruits, vegetables, and legumes are high in fiber. It's important to increase fiber intake gradually to avoid bloating and gas. Diet plays a crucial role in managing diverticulitis by influencing the frequency and severity of flare-ups.

However, some foods can make symptoms worse and should be avoided or limited. These include processed foods high in fats and sugars, which can aggravate digestive discomfort and inflammation. Dairy products and red meat can also make symptoms worse for some people. Staying properly hydrated is also important to help with digestion and soften stools.

Probiotics, which can be found in yogurt and fermented foods, can help with gut health and reduce the likelihood of flare-ups.

WHICH MEALS OUGHT TO BE AVOIDED IF I HAVE DIVERTICULITIS?

Red meat and dairy products, especially those high in fat, may also be problematic for some people as they can be harder to digest and may worsen abdominal discomfort. These foods are important to avoid when managing diverticulitis because they can aggravate symptoms and possibly cause flare-ups. These foods include highly processed foods like fast food, fried items, and sugary snacks.

Furthermore, it's common advice to avoid foods that have small seeds or nuts, such as popcorn, strawberries, and raspberries, because of worries that these tiny particles could become lodged in diverticula and cause irritation or infection; however, tolerance varies and some individuals may find they can tolerate these foods in moderation.

In the end, it's important to collaborate closely with a healthcare provider or registered dietitian to create a customized diet plan that supports digestive health and meets individual needs.

CAN I STILL HAVE DESSERTS AND SNACKS?

Diverticulitis management necessitates careful consideration of dietary choices, but moderation is key. Healthy substitutes can help satiate cravings while promoting digestive health; fresh fruits, such as bananas, apples, and berries, are great because of their fiber content and inherent sweetness; Greek yogurt with probiotics offers a satiating snack that promotes gut health; and for chocolate lovers, higher cocoa content dark chocolate has antioxidants and is less sugary than milk chocolate.

Desserts can be tasty and nutritious when made at home with whole grains and natural sweeteners like honey or maple syrup; baking with oats or whole wheat flour adds fiber, and adding fruits (like baked apples or poached pears) naturally sweetens without the need for added sugars; it's important to pay attention to your body's signals and observe how different foods affect symptoms, making necessary adjustments to maintain overall well-being and digestive comfort.

HOW CAN I MAKE A BALANCED MEAL PLAN?

Diverticulitis meal plans should incorporate a range of nutrient-dense foods while avoiding triggers that could lead to flare-ups. To start, emphasize foods high in fiber, such as whole grains (brown rice, whole wheat pasta), fresh produce (leafy greens, carrots, and berries), and legumes (chickpeas, lentils, and chickpeas). These foods support digestive health and regular bowel movements.

Include healthy fats from sources like olive oil, avocados, and nuts, which provide essential nutrients without adding to digestive discomfort. Plan meals that include lean proteins like poultry, fish, and tofu, which are easier to digest than red meats.

Cook by baking, grilling, or steaming instead of frying, which can add unnecessary fats. Stay hydrated throughout the day by drinking lots of water, which helps soften stools and supports overall digestive function.

Plan snacks that include fresh fruits, raw vegetables with hummus, or whole-grain crackers with low-fat cheese to maintain energy levels between meals. By focusing on nutrient-dense foods and mindful eating habits, you can create a meal plan that supports digestive wellness and lowers the risk of diverticulitis flare-ups. Experiment with herbs and spices instead of using excessive salt or high-fat sauces to keep meals interesting and flavorful.

www.ingramcontent.com/pod-product-compliance
Lightning Source LLC
Chambersburg PA
CBHW071841210526
45479CB00001B/243